COMPLETE JUICING WEIGHT LOSS RECIPES COOKBOOK

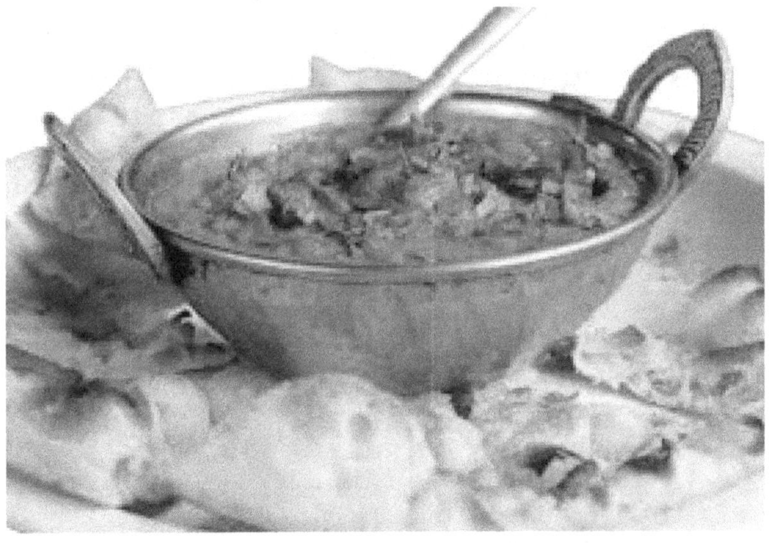

A Comprehensive Guide to Transform Your Body and Boost Health with Nutrient-Rich Recipes, Detox Strategies, and a 4-Week Meal Plan for Natural Weight

Isabelle Hartley

OTHER BOOKS BY THIS AUTHOR

1. <u>GASTROPARESIS DIET RECIPES COOKBOOK</u>
2. <u>HIGH CALORIES DIET COOKBOOK</u>
3. <u>DIET FOR WOMEN OVER FORTY</u>
4. <u>HASHIMOTO RECIPES COOKBOOK</u>
5. <u>JUICING RECIPES FOR CANCER</u>
6. <u>IVF DIET COOKBOOK FOR BEGINNERS</u>
7. <u>LOW SUGAR DIET GUIDE FOR BEGINNERS</u>
8. <u>RAW FOODS RECIPES COOKBOOK</u>
9. <u>SMOOTHIES RECIPES FOR ANTI-INFLAMMATION</u>
10. <u>MEDITERRANEAN DIET FOR PREGNANT WOMEN</u>

TABLE OF CONTENTS

Introduction

In a world saturated with fad diets and quick fixes, Sarah's journey to weight loss stands out as a testament to the transformative power of juicing. Battling with excess weight for years, Sarah decided to embrace a healthier lifestyle by incorporating juicing into her daily routine. Little did she know, this decision would become the cornerstone of her remarkable success story.

Sarah began her juicing journey with a simple goal: to nourish her body with the vital nutrients it craved. Armed with a juicer and a variety of fresh fruits and vegetables, she embarked on a flavorful adventure that would redefine her relationship with food. The first week was a revelation – the vibrant colors and refreshing tastes of her homemade juices replaced the dull monotony of processed snacks.

As the days turned into weeks, Sarah not only noticed a change in her energy levels but also witnessed the numbers on the scale steadily decreasing. The natural detoxifying properties of the nutrient-rich juices were working wonders for her metabolism, and she found herself shedding pounds without feeling deprived or hungry. The fiber from the fruits and vegetables kept her satisfied, curbing cravings for unhealthy snacks.

What started as a quest for weight loss evolved into a holistic transformation. Sarah's skin glowed with newfound radiance, and her overall well-being improved. The journey wasn't without its challenges – adapting to this lifestyle required commitment and perseverance. Yet, the tangible results fueled her determination.

Sarah's success story isn't just about losing weight; it's about embracing a sustainable, health-focused lifestyle. Juicing became more than a routine; it became a source of empowerment and self-discovery. Sarah's journey inspires others to view weight loss not as a quick fix but as a harmonious journey towards nourishing the body, one delicious sip at a time.

Chapter 1

In a world inundated with weight loss trends and quick-fix solutions, the concept of juicing has emerged as a refreshing and effective approach to shedding those extra pounds while nourishing the body from within. The "Juicing for Weight Loss" journey is not just about counting calories; it's a transformative exploration into the vibrant realm of natural, nutrient-dense elixirs that hold the potential to reshape both body and lifestyle.

At its core, juicing for weight loss harnesses the power of whole fruits and vegetables, extracting their essential vitamins, minerals, and antioxidants in liquid form. This liquid gold becomes a potent ally in the pursuit of a healthier, leaner self. The philosophy behind juicing is not one of deprivation but of abundance – flooding the body with the vital nutrients it craves, fostering a sense of fullness, and naturally curbing cravings for less nutritious options.

As we delve into this journey, we will unravel the science behind juicing, exploring how it jumpstarts metabolism, supports natural detoxification, and ignites sustainable weight loss. Beyond the physical aspects, juicing embraces the principle that healthy habits should be a joyous experience, not a daunting task. The symphony of colors, flavors, and aromas in each carefully crafted juice recipe transforms the act of nourishing oneself into a daily celebration of well-being.

This guide seeks to be more than just a compilation of recipes; it is a roadmap for those embarking on the juicing expedition. From selecting the right ingredients to understanding the nuances of various juicing techniques, we will unravel the secrets to success. So, let the juicer become your ally, the fruits and vegetables your accomplices, and embark on a journey where weight loss and well-being harmoniously coexist in each revitalizing sip.

Chapter 2

Weight loss is a multifaceted journey that transcends the mere numbers on a scale; it is a complex interplay of physical, mental, and lifestyle factors that collectively influence one's ability to achieve and sustain a healthier body weight. Understanding the intricacies of weight loss involves navigating through a myriad of factors, from dietary choices and physical activity to psychological aspects and metabolic nuances.

The Physiology of Weight Loss:

At its core, weight loss revolves around the basic principle of achieving a caloric deficit – expending more calories than consumed. This fundamental concept underscores the importance of diet and exercise in any weight loss endeavor. The body, as an intricate machine, responds to this energy imbalance by tapping into stored fat reserves for fuel. However, the journey isn't as simple as calories in versus calories out; the types of calories consumed play a crucial role.

Nutrient-dense foods, rich in vitamins, minerals, and fiber, not only contribute to overall health but also support sustainable weight loss. Incorporating a variety of fruits, vegetables, lean proteins, and whole grains provides the body with essential nutrients while promoting a feeling of fullness. On the contrary, a diet high in processed foods and refined sugars may lead to rapid spikes and crashes in blood sugar levels, contributing to increased cravings and overeating.

The Role of Physical Activity:

While dietary choices lay the foundation for weight loss, physical activity acts as a catalyst. Exercise not only burns calories but also enhances metabolism, making the body more efficient in utilizing energy. Moreover, regular physical activity promotes muscle development, which in turn contributes to increased calorie expenditure even at rest. The synergy between a balanced diet and consistent exercise forms the cornerstone of a successful weight loss strategy.

Psychological Aspects:

Beyond the physiological dimensions, the psychological facets of weight loss are equally pivotal. Emotional eating, stress, and mental well-being can significantly impact one's ability to adhere to a weight loss regimen. Understanding the triggers for overeating and developing healthier coping mechanisms are essential elements of a sustainable weight loss journey. Additionally, cultivating a positive mindset and setting realistic goals can foster resilience in the face of challenges.

Metabolic Variability:

Individual metabolic rates vary, influencing how efficiently the body processes and burns calories. Factors such as age, genetics, and hormonal fluctuations contribute to this metabolic variability. While some individuals may experience rapid weight loss with seemingly minimal effort, others may find the process more gradual. Recognizing and respecting these individual differences is crucial in tailoring a weight loss approach that aligns with one's unique metabolic profile.

Fad Diets vs. Sustainable Practices:

The weight loss landscape is rife with fad diets promising quick results through drastic restrictions or peculiar food combinations. While these approaches may yield temporary weight loss, they often lack sustainability and may compromise nutritional balance. Sustainable weight loss involves adopting lifestyle changes that can be maintained in the long run. It's about fostering a harmonious relationship with food, finding joy in physical activity, and prioritizing overall well-being.

Support Systems and Accountability:

Embarking on a weight loss journey can be challenging, and having a support system can make a significant difference. Whether it's friends, family, or a professional, sharing the experience with others provides encouragement, accountability, and a sense of community. Engaging in weight loss programs, joining fitness classes, or working with a nutritionist can offer guidance and structure, enhancing the likelihood of success.

Plateaus and Adaptability:

Weight loss is rarely a linear process; plateaus and fluctuations are common. Understanding that the body may reach periods of stasis and adapting strategies accordingly is essential. This may involve modifying exercise routines, adjusting caloric intake, or exploring new dietary approaches. The ability to adapt to changing circumstances and persist through plateaus is a hallmark of successful long-term weight management.

Health Implications:

Beyond aesthetic motivations, weight loss holds profound implications for overall health. Excess body weight is associated with a higher risk of various health conditions, including cardiovascular diseases, diabetes, and certain cancers. Achieving and maintaining a healthy weight can mitigate these risks and contribute to improved longevity and quality of life. Weight loss isn't just about fitting into a smaller dress size; it's a commitment to nurturing the body for optimal health and vitality.

In the intricate tapestry of weight loss, each thread represents a unique aspect – from the physiological intricacies of metabolism to the psychological nuances of behavior. It's a journey that goes beyond the superficial pursuit of a number on the scale; it's about cultivating a holistic approach to well-being. A successful weight loss journey involves a commitment to sustainable practices, an understanding of individual variability, and a resilient mindset capable of navigating the complexities of change. Ultimately, the pursuit of weight loss is a dynamic and personal endeavor that, when approached with intention and balance, can lead to transformative outcomes, not just in physical appearance but in overall health and vitality.

Chapter 3

Getting Started with Juicing

Embarking on the journey of juicing for weight loss is an exciting and health-conscious decision. To kickstart this endeavor, it's crucial to lay the foundation with a thoughtful approach to getting started.

Selecting the Right Juicer:

Investing in a quality juicer is the first step. Two common types are centrifugal and cold-press (masticating) juicers. Centrifugal juicers are faster but may generate more heat, potentially affecting nutrient retention. Cold-press juicers operate at lower speeds, preserving more nutrients but are generally slower. Choosing the right juicer depends on personal preferences and priorities.

Choosing Fresh Ingredients:

The essence of juicing lies in the freshness of ingredients. Opt for a colorful array of fruits and vegetables, ensuring a mix of vitamins, minerals, and antioxidants. Organic produce is ideal to minimize exposure to pesticides. Experiment with a variety of ingredients to discover flavor combinations that both satisfy the taste buds and promote weight loss.

Basic Juicing Techniques:

Understanding basic juicing techniques ensures optimal results. Wash and prep ingredients, removing seeds and peels as needed. Rotate ingredients to balance flavors and maximize nutritional diversity. Be mindful of the sugar content in fruits, and consider incorporating more vegetables than fruits for lower calorie content.

Creating Balanced Recipes:

Crafting balanced juice recipes involves considering both flavor profiles and nutritional benefits. Incorporate leafy greens for vitamins and minerals, citrus fruits for a burst of freshness, and a touch of sweetness from low-sugar fruits. Adding herbs like mint or parsley can enhance both taste and detoxifying properties.

Gradual Integration into Routine:

Introduce juicing gradually into daily routines. Begin with one juice a day, perhaps as a replacement for a snack. This allows the body to adjust to increased nutrient intake. Over time, as the palate adapts to the natural sweetness of fresh juices, cravings for processed snacks may diminish.

By carefully selecting the right juicer, choosing fresh ingredients, mastering basic techniques, creating balanced recipes, and gradually integrating juicing into daily life, one sets the stage for a successful and sustainable journey toward weight loss and improved well-being. Juicing becomes not just a dietary choice but a flavorful and nourishing ritual that supports the body's natural ability to shed excess weight.

Essential Juicing Techniques

Mastering essential juicing techniques is key to extracting maximum benefits from your juicing for weight loss journey. These techniques not only enhance the flavor and quality of your juices but also contribute to preserving vital nutrients for optimal health.

Cold Press vs. Centrifugal Juicing:

Understanding the fundamental difference between cold-press (masticating) and centrifugal juicers is crucial. Cold-press juicers operate at lower speeds, minimizing heat generation and preserving more nutrients. This method is ideal for those seeking the utmost nutritional value in their juices. On the other hand, centrifugal juicers work at higher speeds and are faster but may generate more heat, potentially impacting nutrient retention. The choice between the two depends on individual priorities.

Blending for Maximum Nutrient Retention:

While traditional juicing extracts liquid from fruits and vegetables, blending involves keeping the whole produce, including the fiber. This method ensures that the fiber, which aids in digestion and provides a feeling of fullness, is retained in the final product. Blending is an excellent technique for those aiming to incorporate the benefits of both fiber and liquid nutrients into their diet.

Balancing Ingredients:

Achieving a harmonious balance of ingredients is an art in juicing. Incorporate a mix of fruits and vegetables to obtain a broad spectrum of vitamins, minerals, and antioxidants. Leafy greens, such as kale and spinach, are excellent additions for their nutritional density. Strike a balance between sweet and savory elements, ensuring a satisfying and palatable experience with each sip.

Understanding Cold Storage and Shelf Life:

Freshness is paramount in juicing. Consuming juices immediately ensures optimal nutrient intake. However, if storing for later use, consider cold storage in airtight containers to minimize nutrient degradation. Recognize that some juices may separate over time; a quick shake before consumption can restore consistency.

Experimenting with Texture and Consistency:

Explore various textures and consistencies by adjusting the quantity of water or ice added to your juices. Some prefer a thicker, smoothie-like consistency, while others opt for a more liquid form. Personalizing the texture enhances the overall juicing experience, making it a tailored and enjoyable aspect of your weight loss journey.

By mastering these essential juicing techniques, you elevate your juicing experience from a simple beverage preparation to a holistic approach that maximizes nutrient retention, supports weight loss goals, and promotes overall well-being. Juicing becomes a skillful art, empowering you to create flavorful and nutritionally potent concoctions that contribute to a healthier lifestyle.

7-Day Juicing Challenge

Embarking on a 7-day juicing challenge is a transformative and invigorating experience, propelling individuals toward their weight loss goals while infusing the body with a burst of essential nutrients. This structured challenge offers a week-long immersion into the world of vibrant flavors, varied textures, and unparalleled health benefits.

Day 1-2: Green Kickstart

Begin the challenge with nutrient-packed green juices. Incorporate kale, spinach, cucumber, and a touch of lemon for a refreshing start. These leafy greens provide a powerhouse of vitamins and minerals while kickstarting your metabolism.

Day 3-4: Citrus Revival

Transition into a citrus-infused phase to revitalize your taste buds. Oranges, grapefruits, and lemons not only add zesty flavors but also contribute to detoxification and hydration. These juices provide a burst of vitamin C, supporting immune function.

Day 5-6: Berry Bliss

Introduce antioxidant-rich berries like blueberries and raspberries. These vibrant fruits not only add a sweet and tart dimension to your juices but also combat oxidative stress, promoting overall well-being. Mix them with greens for a delightful fusion.

Day 7: Tropical Farewell

Conclude the challenge with tropical flavors like pineapple, mango, and coconut water. These juices add a tropical twist to your palate while providing essential nutrients. Pineapple, in particular, contains bromelain, an enzyme known for its digestion-aiding properties.

Tips for Success:

Hydration is Key: Ensure you stay hydrated throughout the challenge by drinking water alongside your juices.

- Listen to Your Body: If hunger strikes, consider incorporating a small, healthy snack to maintain energy levels.

- Variety is Essential: Experiment with different ingredients to keep the challenge exciting and diverse.

- Post-Challenge Transition: Gradually reintroduce solid foods after the challenge, focusing on whole, nutritious options.

Chapter 4

Benefits of the 7-Day Juicing Challenge:

Weight Loss Kickstart: The challenge provides a caloric deficit, aiding in initial weight loss.

Increased Nutrient Intake: Flood your body with essential vitamins, minerals, and antioxidants for improved overall health.

Improved Digestion: The fiber in some juices and the hydration from others contribute to digestive well-being.

Enhanced Energy Levels: The natural sugars from fruits provide sustained energy without the crashes associated with processed sugars.

The 7-day juicing challenge is not just a dietary endeavor; it's a rejuvenating experience that resets the palate, promotes mindful nutrition, and lays the foundation for sustained well-being. As participants savor each flavorful sip, they embark on a journey towards a healthier lifestyle, armed with newfound knowledge and a refreshed perspective on the benefits of juicing for weight loss.

Juicing Recipes for Weight Loss

Here are 10 delicious juicing recipes tailored for weight loss, featuring a mix of vibrant fruits and nutrient-packed vegetables:

1. Green Goddess Detox Juice:

Ingredients:

- 2 cups spinach
- 1 cucumber
- 2 celery stalks
- 1 green apple
- 1/2 lemon (peeled)

Preparation:

1. Wash all ingredients thoroughly.
2. Cut them into smaller pieces for easier juicing.
3. Feed the ingredients through your juicer.
4. Stir well and pour over ice for a refreshing detox drink.

2. Citrus Slim Down Elixir:

Ingredients:

- 2 oranges (peeled)
- 1 grapefruit (peeled)
- 1 lemon (peeled)
- 1-inch ginger root

Preparation:

1. Peel the citrus fruits and chop into manageable pieces.
2. Add the ginger for a metabolism boost.
3. Juice all ingredients together.
4. Pour into a glass and enjoy the zesty freshness.
5. 3. Berry Blast Fat Burner:

Ingredients:

- 1 cup blueberries
- 1 cup strawberries
- 1/2 cup raspberries
- 1/2 cup blackberries

- 1 apple

Preparation:

1. Wash and prepare the berries and apple.
2. Juice all the ingredients together.
3. This antioxidant-rich juice is a flavorful way to boost metabolism.

4. Pineapple Paradise Slimming Juice:

Ingredients:

- 2 cups pineapple chunks
- 1 cucumber
- 1 green apple
- 1/2 lime (peeled)

Preparation:

1. Peel and chop the pineapple, cucumber, and apple.
2. Juice all ingredients.
3. The tropical flavors make this a delightful weight loss elixir.

5. Beetroot Boost Juice:

Ingredients:

- 1 medium-sized beetroot (peeled)
- 2 carrots
- 1 apple
- 1-inch ginger root

Preparation:

1. Prepare and chop all ingredients.
2. Juice them together.
3. Beetroot adds a rich color and nutrients to this energizing blend.

6. Mango Tango Fat Burner:

Ingredients:

- 2 cups mango chunks
- 1 orange (peeled)
- 1/2 lime (peeled)
- 1 cucumber

Preparation:

- Peel and chop the mango, orange, and cucumber.
- Juice all the ingredients together.
- Enjoy the tropical flavors with a metabolism-boosting twist.

7. Spinach Celery Cleanse:

Ingredients:

- 2 cups spinach
- 3 celery stalks
- 1 cucumber
- 1 green apple
- 1/2 lemon (peeled)

Preparation:

1. Wash and chop all ingredients.
2. Juice together for a refreshing and cleansing green drink.

8. Carrot Ginger Zinger:

Ingredients:

1.   4 large carrots
2.   1 orange (peeled)
3.   1-inch ginger root

Preparation:

1.   Wash and prepare the carrots and orange.
2.   Juice them along with the ginger for a zesty kick.

9. Blueberry Bliss Lemonade:

Ingredients:

- 1 cup blueberries
- 1/2 cup strawberries
- 2 lemons (peeled)

Preparation:

1.   Wash the berries and lemons.

2. Juice them together for a delightful berry-infused lemonade.

10. Kale and Pineapple Power Punch:

Ingredients:

- 2 cups kale
- 2 cups pineapple chunks
- 1 green apple
- 1/2 lemon (peeled)

Preparation:

1. Wash and chop the kale, pineapple, and apple.
2. Juice all the ingredients for a nutrient-packed power punch.

Remember to adjust the quantities based on your taste preferences and the size of your juicer. Enjoy these flavorful and nutrient-rich juices as part of your weight loss journey.

CONCLUSION

In conclusion, juicing for weight loss is not merely a dietary approach; it is a holistic lifestyle transformation that blends the goodness of nature with the pursuit of optimal well-being. Through a symphony of flavors, essential nutrients, and mindful nutrition, juicing provides a sustainable and enjoyable path toward shedding excess weight and embracing a healthier version of oneself.

The 7-day juicing challenge serves as a testament to the versatility and efficacy of this approach. From the detoxifying Green Goddess to the refreshing Berry Blast, each juice offers a unique blend of vitamins, minerals, and antioxidants that nourish the body and support weight loss goals. The interplay of flavors not only tantalizes the taste buds but also fuels the body with the energy needed for an active and vibrant lifestyle.

Beyond the physiological benefits, juicing fosters a mindful connection to what we consume. It encourages a departure from processed, calorie-dense foods and invites a return to the simplicity and purity of natural ingredients. As we savor the vibrant hues of each concoction, we reconnect with the essence of nourishing our bodies from the inside out.

So, dear reader, let this be not just a fleeting foray into juicing but a commitment to a lifestyle that prioritizes health and vitality. Embrace the journey, relish the diverse flavors, and witness the transformative power of juicing unfold in your life. As you adopt and adapt to this enriching dietary practice, remember that every sip is a step towards a healthier you. Let the vibrant colors in your glass be a reminder of the colorful and vibrant life that awaits you on this juicing journey. Cheers to a healthier, happier you!

Contact Us

Dear Reader,

If you have any questions, need further clarification, or require assistance with any aspect of the book, please do not hesitate to reach out to me. I am more than happy to provide additional insights, address your queries, or simply engage in a meaningful discussion.

Feel free to contact me at: IsabelleHartleyBooks@gmail.com. Your feedback and inquiries are always welcome.

FREE 30 DAYS MEAL PLANNER

FREE 30Days Meal Planner, a priceless extra to get you started on the path to a more organized and healthy living. This meticulously curated planner is made to make meal planning easier, save you time, and help you meet your nutritional objectives. Prepare to enjoy the advantages of this wonderful resource!

DAILY MEAL PLANNER

Day: ....

BREAKFAST

____

____

LUNCH

____

____

DINNER

____

____

INGREDIENTS NEEDED

☐ _____________________________________

☐ _____________________________________

☐ _____________________________________

☐ _____________________________________

DAILY MEAL PLANNER

Day: ....

BREAKFAST

____

____

LUNCH

____

____

DINNER

____

____

INGREDIENTS NEEDED

☐ _______________________________________

☐ _______________________________________

☐ _______________________________________

☐ _______________________________________

DAILY MEAL PLANNER

Day: ....

BREAKFAST

____

____

LUNCH

____

____

DINNER

____

____

INGREDIENTS NEEDED

☐ _______________________________________

☐ _______________________________________

☐ _______________________________________

☐ _______________________________________

DAILY MEAL PLANNER

Day: ....

BREAKFAST

____

____

LUNCH

____

____

DINNER

____

____

INGREDIENTS NEEDED

☐ ___________________________________

☐ ___________________________________

☐ ___________________________________

☐ ___________________________________

DAILY MEAL PLANNER

Day: ....

BREAKFAST

____

____

LUNCH

____

____

DINNER

____

____

INGREDIENTS NEEDED

☐ _____________________________________

☐ _____________________________________

☐ _____________________________________

☐ _____________________________________

DAILY MEAL PLANNER

Day: ....

BREAKFAST

____

____

LUNCH

____

____

DINNER

____

____

INGREDIENTS NEEDED

☐ _______________________________________

☐ _______________________________________

☐ _______________________________________

☐ _______________________________________

DAILY MEAL PLANNER

Day: ....

BREAKFAST

____

____

LUNCH

____

____

DINNER

____

____

INGREDIENTS NEEDED

- ☐ _______________________________________
- ☐ _______________________________________
- ☐ _______________________________________
- ☐ _______________________________________

DAILY MEAL PLANNER

Day: ....

BREAKFAST

LUNCH

DINNER

INGREDIENTS NEEDED

- [ ]
- [ ]
- [ ]
- [ ]

DAILY MEAL PLANNER

Day:

BREAKFAST

LUNCH

DINNER

INGREDIENTS NEEDED

- [ ]
- [ ]
- [ ]
- [ ]

DAILY MEAL PLANNER

Day: ....

BREAKFAST

____

____

LUNCH

____

____

DINNER

____

____

INGREDIENTS NEEDED

- ☐ _______________________________
- ☐ _______________________________
- ☐ _______________________________
- ☐ _______________________________

DAILY MEAL PLANNER

Day: _______________________________

BREAKFAST

____

____

LUNCH

____

____

DINNER

____

____

INGREDIENTS NEEDED

☐ _______________________________

☐ _______________________________

☐ _______________________________

☐ _______________________________

DAILY MEAL PLANNER

Day: ....

BREAKFAST

LUNCH

DINNER

INGREDIENTS NEEDED

- [ ]
- [ ]
- [ ]
- [ ]

DAILY MEAL PLANNER

Day: ....

BREAKFAST

____

____

LUNCH

____

____

DINNER

____

____

INGREDIENTS NEEDED

☐ _______________________________________

☐ _______________________________________

☐ _______________________________________

☐ _______________________________________

DAILY MEAL PLANNER

Day: ....

BREAKFAST

____

____

LUNCH

____

____

DINNER

____

____

INGREDIENTS NEEDED

☐ _______________________________

☐ _______________________________

☐ _______________________________

☐ _______________________________

DAILY MEAL PLANNER

Day:

BREAKFAST

LUNCH

DINNER

INGREDIENTS NEEDED

- ☐
- ☐
- ☐
- ☐

DAILY MEAL PLANNER

Day: ....

BREAKFAST

____

____

LUNCH

____

____

DINNER

____

____

INGREDIENTS NEEDED

☐ ____

☐ ____

☐ ____

☐ ____

DAILY MEAL PLANNER

Day: ....

BREAKFAST

LUNCH

DINNER

INGREDIENTS NEEDED

- ☐
- ☐
- ☐
- ☐

DAILY MEAL PLANNER

Day: ....

BREAKFAST

____

____

LUNCH

____

____

DINNER

____

____

INGREDIENTS NEEDED

☐ _______________________________

☐ _______________________________

☐ _______________________________

☐ _______________________________

DAILY MEAL PLANNER

Day:

BREAKFAST

LUNCH

DINNER

INGREDIENTS NEEDED

DAILY MEAL PLANNER

Day:

BREAKFAST

LUNCH

DINNER

INGREDIENTS NEEDED

- [ ]
- [ ]
- [ ]
- [ ]

DAILY MEAL PLANNER

Day: ....

BREAKFAST

____

____

LUNCH

____

____

DINNER

____

____

INGREDIENTS NEEDED

☐ _______________________________________

☐ _______________________________________

☐ _______________________________________

☐ _______________________________________

DAILY MEAL PLANNER

Day: ....

BREAKFAST

____

____

LUNCH

____

____

DINNER

____

____

INGREDIENTS NEEDED

☐ _____________________________________

☐ _____________________________________

☐ _____________________________________

☐ _____________________________________

DAILY MEAL PLANNER

Day: ....

BREAKFAST

____

____

LUNCH

____

____

DINNER

____

____

INGREDIENTS NEEDED

☐ ____

☐ ____

☐ ____

☐ ____

DAILY MEAL PLANNER

Day: ....

BREAKFAST

LUNCH

DINNER

INGREDIENTS NEEDED

- ☐
- ☐
- ☐
- ☐

DAILY MEAL PLANNER

Day: ....

BREAKFAST

____

____

LUNCH

____

____

DINNER

____

____

INGREDIENTS NEEDED

☐ _______________________________________

☐ _______________________________________

☐ _______________________________________

☐ _______________________________________

DAILY MEAL PLANNER

Day: ....

BREAKFAST

____

____

LUNCH

____

____

DINNER

____

____

INGREDIENTS NEEDED

☐ _____________________________________

☐ _____________________________________

☐ _____________________________________

☐ _____________________________________

DAILY MEAL PLANNER

Day:

BREAKFAST

LUNCH

DINNER

INGREDIENTS NEEDED

DAILY MEAL PLANNER

Day: ....

BREAKFAST

____

____

LUNCH

____

____

DINNER

____

____

INGREDIENTS NEEDED

- [ ] _______________________________________
- [ ] _______________________________________
- [ ] _______________________________________
- [ ] _______________________________________

DAILY MEAL PLANNER

Day: ....

BREAKFAST

LUNCH

DINNER

INGREDIENTS NEEDED

DAILY MEAL PLANNER

Day: ....

BREAKFAST

____

____

LUNCH

____

____

DINNER

____

____

INGREDIENTS NEEDED

☐ _______________________________

☐ _______________________________

☐ _______________________________

☐ _______________________________

DAILY MEAL PLANNER

Day: ....

BREAKFAST

____

____

LUNCH

____

____

DINNER

____

____

INGREDIENTS NEEDED

☐ _______________________________________

☐ _______________________________________

☐ _______________________________________

☐ _______________________________________